The Anti-Aging Guide To Aging Backwards

Learn To Age Well, Age Gracefully And Make It The Happiest Time Of Your Life

By Michele Gilbert

Visit My Amazon Author Page

Table of contents

Introduction

I want to thank you and congratulate you for downloading the book, *"The Anti-Aging Guide To Aging Backwards"*.

This book contains proven steps and strategies on how to slow down your biological clock and even turn it back.

You probably picked this book up because you've already had 'that' moment, the one where you looked in the mirror and for a second you didn't know who that person was. We've all had that moment, and they happen more often after forty. In your head you are young and blithe, but something unnerving is happening to the outer casket. Sometimes it is happening ahead of schedule, the alarming phenomenon of premature aging.

We all want to look, act and feel good for our age. We want to look younger than our friends. We'd like people to be surprised (in a good way) when they learn how old we actually are!

The minute I find out how to wave a wand and make it happen overnight, I'll tell you. I promise. But this book will tell you how turn the clock back on your appearance, slow the aging process down, and enjoy good looks and vitality in the future; effectively, age backwards.

Thanks again for downloading this book, I hope you enjoy it!

Introducing the concept of aging backwards:

There's a lot of pressure on looking young these days. Photo-shopped models, every flaw and blemish removed from their photographs, are presented as normal. Actors and TV presenters insist on special filters being used on cameras. Before and after 'shock' photos show a thirty-year-old publicity shot of a celebrity, next to a candid camera pic that must make them want to eat their own livers in rage and frustration. The message is loud and clear. If you don't look wonderful, you're a has-been.

Of course that is media in-house warfare, and ridiculous, and everyone knows it is ridiculous. Still, the fact is that we are statistically likely to live longer than our grandparents did. We have access to better food, and better health facilities, and age is not the absolute number it was.

You are as young as you feel, and you don't feel as young as you would like to feel, which is why you bought this book.

Whatever age you are, forty-something and all the way up, you want to reverse the damage your younger self did, make the most of what you are now, and bring the aging process down to a crawl so that instead of aging *faster* than you should, you age more *slowly*.

Just a word, here, about realistic expectations. It *will* take up to a month to feel and see a real difference (although there are some quick fix options for special occasions) and several months for real improvement. However, real improvement is *guaranteed*.

Your body, by the way, is 100% behind you on this. We're told the human body is designed to live around 120 years. Bits of us are capable of more—a healthy heart, for instance, can live much longer than the body it powers—yet young athletes can have heart attacks. We are potentially capable of being healthy and vigorous for a century. You just need to find out how.

CHAPTER 1
The causes of accelerated aging

Sun damage

The sun is vital to our health, but no-one, no matter their colour, can assume their skin needs no assistance. The lighter your skin, the more protection you need. From this *minute* on, use at least a Factor 15 cream every day on any exposed skin. Your skin has had enough sun. Protect it.

Smoking

Smokers will always look older, because smoking roughens facial skin and puts deeper lines around the mouth. There are ways of minimising the damage to your appearance, but for now make the following immediate changes: smoke outside. Don't smoke the cigarette right to the filter. Consider getting a holder. Cut down.

Poor diet

The older you are, the more you need to give your body the nutrients it needs to be strong and healthy. The chances are that even if you believe you have a healthy diet, you're not eating the most effective foods.

Stress

The main way that stress affects appearance is obvious lack of care: you don't have time to spend on yourself. Lack of care, though, affects more than your appearance. Living on adrenaline affects your outer appearance, but also affects your long-term health and vitality.

Lack of Exercise

Your muscles lose tone, your skin will start to sag, you lose stamina, and energy and strength dwindle. Your posture and ease of movement can affect your appearance by twenty years either way, depending on whether you bounce or shuffle.

Trauma

Heart attacks, cancer, strokes, pneumonia and serious accidents are all traumatic and affect appearance. How often have you heard that so-and-so has never been the same since? It's hard: but you can get back.

Pain

Aches and pains are part of the aging process, and pain is debilitating. However, don't accept it as inevitable. Track down the cause and deal with it.

Loss of fun

Laughter is the best medicine, and it certainly keeps you young. Life can seem less amusing as you get older. Recover the fun.

CHAPTER 2
Slow down biological aging

In this chapter we'll look at the key factors above, expand on some, and introduce others. What you should be eating, for health and energy, has its own chapter. Working towards a sound mind in a healthy body also has its own chapter. In this one we will be addressing the whole plan of action.

To slow down the aging process, we tackle it on several fronts at once. *You want to look good, move well, and feel great.* The key factors are sleeping well, eating effectively, finding an exercise regime you like, and your general appearance. That last isn't just vanity. People react to your appearance and you react to their response. If they see you as tired and older, they will treat you as tired and older and you will *feel* tired and older. You only get one chance to make a first impression. You want to come across as interesting and worth knowing. There's a chapter just on appearance, because it is that important.

Sleeping well

Is the biggest key to health. As you get older, your sleep patterns change. You may find you are sleeping less, and perfectly happy on four hours a night. Or you are going to bed earlier and sleeping ten hours a night and feel great when you wake up. You may vary between the two extremes. As long as you are happy with the sleep you are getting, ignore what people say you 'should' be having. It can be hard, though, when you live with someone who is developing a different sleep pattern and in trying to adjust to each other, you both run into sleep difficulties. Talk it through, and go with what suits you individually.

Remember also that as you get older your sleep needs are in flux. Just because you usually like to go to bed at nine, don't automatically go to bed at nine if you aren't sleepy, or think there must be a problem if you are tired hours earlier than usual. A good night is the start of a good day.

Many people do find that sleep is suddenly becoming elusive. They battle to get to sleep, wake in the early hours of the morning, or feel unrested when they wake up. This can be either because they're ignoring the sleep patterns their body wants, or because of stress. Exercising during the day, with perhaps a last stroll at night, waiting until you feel tired, clearing your mind with pleasant thoughts before you drop off, can all improve your chances of sleeping well. If there is a stress factor, can it be minimized? There's a bit about stress further on. Having a hot drink before you go to bed (chamomile tea is ideal) or reading for ten minutes in bed, can help. Try to avoid relying on sleeping pills.

As you improve your day-time routines and food intake, your nights should improve too. If, though, with all the changes to your lifestyle, you find your nights are getting no better, there are some gentle sleep aids in the chapter on useful additives.

Eating well

Your dietary needs change as you get older. In your twenties and thirties you can pretty much eat anything and keep going. By your forties, certain foods contribute to middle-age spread. By your fifties, there are some foods you no longer tolerate as well as you did. By your sixties, there are foods you have to actively avoid.

Avoid fad diets, especially starvation ones; the older you get, the more vital a proper dietary regime becomes, to avoid premature or accelerated aging.

Push up the amount of protein in your diet. Don't economize on food—buy the best you can afford. There's an old saying we tend to forget; every dollar spent on the table is a dollar less at the doctor.

Get into a habit of eating smaller meals, more often. There are some general all-round vitamins and minerals you need to add in, if you aren't getting them through what you are eating, and they are listed in the chapter on useful additives. The good news is that if you do have some middle-aged spread to shift and re-shape, this dietary advice does that, too.

Managing Stress

Stress is an essential part of healthy living. Without challenges and pressures we would lead very dull and sedentary lives. The body copes very well, as a general rule, and you should find being challenged actually makes you feel invigorated and enthusiastic. It is one reason new retirement can seem a bit traumatic, because of the loss of daily challenges. New retirees soon learn they can choose much more interesting ones.

However, prolonged or unreasonable stress can affect your sleep and your health dramatically. Managing stress is *essential* to slowing down biological aging. Sleeping, exercising and eating properly all contribute to effective stress management. Mental attitude is important. It is easy to feel daunted, as 'stress' is such a buzzword these days, but if you can see it as a positive challenge, you trigger the right hormones to help you deal with it. Telling yourself you can't cope is not going to help. Tell yourself you can find a way to cope.

If your stress is work-related and chronic, with no end in sight, talk to your manager and if there is no alternative, look for other employment. This is *your* life and *your* health. You want them to outlast your job.

If you can change or leave the stressful situation, do so. If you can reduce the impact, do so. At worst, reduce other sources of stress. Stop listening to the news, for example, or getting upset about situations which don't directly affect you, and which you can't change.

A great deal of stress management depends on the situation causing the stress. If it is unavoidable and inescapable—terminal illness in a loved one, for example—share the load. There are support groups everywhere, for everything, even if you have to go online to find them. This is also true for **Trauma**. Recovering a positive mental attitude is your best resource to get you on track for the rest of this book. You are a survivor. Lift your chin and be proud.

Exercise

Exercise is not just running marathons, lifting weights and setting impossible targets. In fact, it shouldn't be, because that can actually accelerate the aging process. Introducing healthy exercise is as simple as walking, climbing stairs, ten minutes in the morning to warm your muscles up for the day, occasional workouts to get your sluggish blood moving and bring a glow to your whole system. Well-managed exercise shouldn't leave you tired afterwards, but revitalized, and with a feeling of well-being. Read the chapter.

Ask those bright-eyed rosy-cheeked couples in their eighties what their secret is. They may be too shy to tell you. If you don't have someone currently in your life, I'm not saying you should start instantly dating, because that in itself can induce stress! But if you do have someone, and aren't making the most of that priceless resource, what a waste. Woo your partner as much as you would woo a new person in your life, because where things were good before, they can be again, and the benefits for you both are lifelong.

Managing Pain

Pain affects sleep, your enjoyment of food, and your ability to exercise, and taking daily pain-killers is not good for your system. Pain ages you, and prolonged pain must be tracked down and dealt with. Regular headaches could mean you need new glasses, for example. We all have occasional aches and twinges, but if your pain persists more than a week, get it checked and sorted. Don't just decide it is a sign of age and resign yourself to it. It will accelerate the aging process if you do.

Relaxation and fun

Make a point of meeting up with friends regularly, no matter how busy your life is. Take up a new hobby, or go along to watch others doing something which interests you. The exercise suggestions in this book are genuinely enjoyable. Play cards, read for fun, watch television shows that make you smile. Learn to say no to invitations which don't interest you at all, and seek out activities which do. Include people who make you feel good, and exclude people who don't, even if you have known them for a very long time. You would be lucky indeed to look forward to everything in your life, but at least minimise the encounters that make you feel bored and depressed.

CHAPTER 3
Looking younger

Everything you've read so far is going to improve your outlook on life, and your general health, and that will show more with every week that passes.

Would you like a quick fix, right now, today, to get you motivated?

- **A haircut.** Consider adding highlights to frame your face, and a layered cut to add bounce.

- **A manicure**. Our hands are the true clue to our age, and you will be working on them a *lot* over the improvement stages, but a manicure improves appearance immediately. Nicely shaped nails, whether buffed or painted, draw attention from the rest of your hand.

- **Whiten your teeth**. Your drugstore will have a paint-on quick-fix. It feels oddly grainy, and your smile won't be blinding, but there will be a definite, confidence-building, difference. (Be warned, red wine and beetroot could turn your smile pink, read the label.)

- **Use eye-whitening eye drops**.

- **Vaseline** is your friend, for the quick fix. Soak your hands in warm water for ten minutes, then gently smooth on Vaseline to trap the moisture for longer. Use a tiny dab of it to sleek your eyebrows and leave a faint highlighting shine on your brow bones. You can even smooth a fine layer on your cheekbones and lips. The trick is not to be sticky, just very slightly shining with health.

- Get fitted for a new **bra**, for an instant improvement to your silhouette. All department stores carry body-shaping **underwear**, take advice and try on different types.

- If this super-quick makeover is for a **special event**, avoid sodium, which can make you retain water, and the gassier vegetables, which can make you bloat, for a couple of days beforehand.

Improving your appearance steadily over time.

Don't stick with a **hairstyle** you've been finding boring-but-easy. If you've been dyeing your hair the same colour for years, stop. Your skin has changed; your colour probably needs to change too. As a general rule, the older you are, the more flattering a softer hair colour is. Discuss options with your hairdresser. You may decide to head towards a completely different style which needs your hair to grow out a bit, and they can start the process with a trim that will start the new shape in the right direction. Give yourself a hot oil treatment at six-to-eight week intervals. Buy a good shampoo. Don't use conditioner every time you wash your hair, it makes it heavy and limp, use it instead every five or six washes. Rinsing your hair in cold water and putting your hairdryer on the cooler setting will give you shinier hair. Brush your hair a hundred times a day for lasting gloss and colour.

Look after your **hands**, and give them twice as much moisturizer as the rest of your body. Have regular manicures, keep your nails looking good, and invest in attractive rings. People *do* notice hands and you can't hide them, so give them something distracting to look at.

An eyebath is a great investment for tired, scratchy eyes. Your drugstore will sell the solution with an eyebath. Do it once a week or as needed.

Whitening your teeth can be done by your dentist, but there are good kits available at drugstores. You don't want blinding white, but yellow or brown teeth are not flattering. Getting them nearer white is very effective for making you look younger. Buy a good toothbrush and replace it regularly.

Book a trip to the dentist especially if you haven't been for a while. Good teeth are essential to good diet. If you aren't chewing your food properly, you aren't getting maximum benefit from it. Go regularly, every six months. By the time you hit your sixties and seventies, you will be either be kicking yourself for skipping the dentist, or grateful for every uncomfortable half hour you ever spent there. The older you are, the more chewing your food properly, and eating slowly, will slow the aging process.

Sun-cream and moisturizer are essential, from this day on and for ever more. As nice as a tan can be, if you rush it, you damage your skin for life. Have a beauty salon spray-tan if you are going on holiday to a sunny place, moisturize every day, use a filtering sun-cream, and build the colour slowly on healthy, happy skin. Never use a sunbed. *Ever.*

Experiment with makeup. Never use a foundation more than two tones away from your own skin-colour, and blend it in well with a damp sponge. If you've used exactly the same make-up for years, it probably doesn't suit your skin these days as well as it did. Reflective makeup is the older woman's friend: a light-reflective primer under your makeup, and lip gloss over your lipstick, are both remarkably effective. Find a good lip-plumper because lips do get a little thinner as we get older. Watch a few YouTube makeovers for ideas.

As a general rule, the older you get, the less makeup you should wear, because heavy or dark makeup on tired skin is very aging. Give yourself facemasks fairly regularly; there are some wonderful ones you can make at home, and some good products across the counter. Spend a little more to get the best available.

Get your eyebrows professionally shaped. If you have light brows and lashes, think about getting them tinted.

Sort out your underwear. If it doesn't fit well, or is uncomfortable, bin it. Your new look starts from the skin up and your underwear should be both working towards your new look and comfortable to wear.

Check your wardrobe. Everything in it should be in a colour and style that flatters you. Hard dramatic colors can be teamed with softer pastels. Soft pink is the most flattering colour of all, especially when worn near the face, but can be insipid; try a soft pink scarf with a favourite outfit rather than wearing pink from top to toe. Good shoes are a must—good looking, and well-fitted.

You will either lose weight or find your body-shape changing, as you follow the diet and exercise suggestions coming up, so don't rush out to invest hugely in new clothes just yet. Buy smart, from now on, so that everything you get works with everything you own already.

Posture. Shuffling as you walk, hunched shoulders, and poor posture, all add years to your age. *Good* posture makes you look years *younger* than your real age. This will happen through exercise, but take advantage if there is someone teaching the Alexander technique near you, because perfect posture has a near-miraculous effect on your respiratory and digestive system as well as your appearance.

Check your bathroom. Time to get rid of harsh detergents, over-aggressive scrubs, and cheap hair-damaging shampoos. Your laundry detergent directly affects your skin—is yours a good one? If your toothbrush and hairbrush have seen better days, replace them with the best you can afford. Get a good set of bathroom scales and weigh yourself at least once a week. Exfoliate regularly, but use a gentle scrub. It's slower, but it won't take off healthy skin with the dead cells!

Check your kitchen. Clear out your freezer and cupboards, and restock from the chapter on food, rather than cramming the new purchases into the same places as the old. You are making a new start and a clear-out is very cathartic.

CHAPTER 4
Eating for health and energy

Your guidelines

The following are guidelines for the rest of your life.

Eat slowly. Chew thoroughly. There's a wide range listed below, but remember, everything in moderation. **Don't eat the same things every day**, repeat favourites after three days. Drink a lot of water, preferably ten minutes before a meal rather than with it. Filtered water is much better than bottled water. One glass of **red wine** is good for you, and so is one cup of **coffee**. Green **tea**, red tea, white tea, and chamomile tea, enjoy freely.

Seasoning is fine (cinnamon is actively good for you) but try to cut back on salt. Even better, switch to sea salt in a grinder.

Avoid processed food. That includes things you have probably considered healthy—soy sauce and commercial fruit juice, to name just two that are heavily marketed as essential to health and wellbeing. The more processed a food is, the fewer nutrients remain, and the more chemicals and preservatives have been added. Chemicals and preservatives are good for keeping food from going bad, but they are not good nutrition.

Anything marked low fat is likely to be higher in sugar. And over-processed, anyway.

Anything grown **cheaply and in bulk** is grown in a kind of chemical dust made up of artificial nutrients and pesticides. Every animal that is raised commercially is fed that same cheap bulk-produced food. We can't escape the chemicals, but we can reduce our intake and therefore boost our health as far as possible. **Buy organic** wherever possible. Even organic foods are not 100% natural but you probably don't have time yourself to grow everything you want to eat. Anyway, picking off bugs by hand would suddenly make you understand why organic farmers had to find a human-friendly solution.

Eat *real* **food** rather than replacements, wherever possible. Raw sugar is better than refined sugar. Refined sugar is better than chemical sweeteners. Butter is better than margarine. Cut down your sugar and butter intake rather than switching.

That may go against everything you have believed for years. However, your body was designed to efficiently interact with the flora and fauna that were naturally available. It will take a while before it can easily metabolize alternatives that are stiff with additives, preservatives, chemicals and artificial nutrients.

Avoid fad diets, and let calorie counting be your servant, not your master. **Tip:** any packaged snack with a shelf-life of months, no matter how beguiling the low calorie count is, should be avoided. Your body, as I said above, is not geared to cope. It will store the entire snack as fat and send up a message saying *hey, still waiting for food here. Feed me.*

So what should you be eating? Three smaller meals a day, high in protein and antioxidants. Three snacks a day (*not* packaged ones), to boost your energy levels in between. If you are about to change from one or two meals a day, remember they will now be much smaller meals. The good news is that the ideal foods are rather nice.

Stocking your pantry

Protein: eggs, oily fish such as salmon, sardines and mackerel, free-range chicken, and organically-raised beef and pork. Protein is not only animal based. Avocado, chickpeas, lentils, kidney beans, nuts, pumpkin seeds and other vegetarian standbys are useful sources.

Dairy – butter, milk, cheese, cream, are all welcome in moderation. Buy organic whenever possible. Greek yoghurt is healthier than most others—compare labels for yourself. Buy natural yoghurt and add your own colors and fruit for favour.

Real honey is one of the miracle foods and a good sweetener. However, commercial honey is produced by putting trays of sugar next to hives and is therefore just bee-digested sugar. Organic honey costs a great deal more. Treat yourself.

Vegetables and salads are filling and good sources of Vitamin C and antioxidants, good news for your skin and your health. Stock up on tomatoes, bell peppers, broccoli, sweet potatoes, spinach (raw in salad is nicer than cooked) and Brussel sprouts in particular. Avocados are laden with skin-improving nutrients. Anything in season grown organically is more than welcome: buy in bulk, chop, blanch and freeze to extend the benefit.

Make your own salad dressings with basics like olive oil and balsamic vinegar; the commercial ones are stiff with 'permitted' preservatives. Mayonnaise is made with oil and egg yolks, both of which are in your diet, and is easy to make if you have a food processor. Don't make a huge batch, it doesn't last very long unless you add a ton of preservatives, which is exactly what you are trying to avoid.

Fruit is a great source of Vitamin C and antioxidants; particularly watermelon, grapefruit, oranges, lemons, limes, guava, strawberries, blueberries, pineapple, mango, grapes, apples and plums. Make a fruit salad and treat yourself to a dollop of organic cream, or Greek yoghurt. Make smoothies. Dried or desiccated fruit, if you do it yourself, is high in concentrated fructose sugar but useful for snacks.

Carbohydrates should largely be covered by your vegetable and salad intake. However, organic brown rice is useful fiber and also a protein source. Potatoes, especially new potatoes in their skins, ditto. Pasta should be kept to a minimum; it is all too easy to slip into using it as 90% of your meal, and there are no benefits to you in doing that, especially as it is often made from commercially-grown genetically-modified wheat which was developed to build rapid bulk in livestock. Unless, of course, you are looking for rapid bulk.

Snacks

A banana, although not listed as a skin-improving fruit, has other excellent qualities and makes an ideal snack. Another ideal snack is slicing an apple and eating it with slices of hard cheese. The combination is delicious and surprisingly filling. Don't cheat and use that oddly rubbery processed cheese, buy organic hard cheese and slice your own.

Hard-boiled eggs and slices of cold chicken and cold meats are also handy snacks.

Nuts are excellent snacks, particularly **almonds and peanuts.** Buy them in their shells where possible. Avoid the salted ones.

Occasional treats

Coffee, red wine, and dark chocolate are all actively good for you if taken in strict moderation.

Drinks

Drink a lot of water to brighten your skin and sluice your system. Ideally, drink before a meal, rather than during, for maximum digestion efficiency. A cup of coffee a day is beneficial. Tea is good, and the white, red and green teas are very good. A glass of red wine in the evening aids digestion. Chamomile tea before bedtime aids restful sleep.

Alcohol generally, especially spirits, does increase facial redness and capillary damage, which accelerates the appearance of aging. Cut it back, or cut it out, to slow down the process.

Your day

Breakfast Don't skip breakfast. Within an hour of waking, your body needs fuel, and keeping it properly fuelled all day will put a spring in your step and improve your health overall. The best breakfast for slow-burning energy, especially in cold weather, is oatmeal porridge, served with cream and a drizzle of real honey, but it isn't to everyone's taste and making it properly takes time. Some people do far better on a protein breakfast, and it can be the quickest option, if you keep cold meat, hardboiled eggs or cheese, on hand. Fruit is not the best start to the day, as it spikes your blood sugar. Eating breakfast is one of the most important weapons in the war against accelerated aging.

Mid-morning snack can be as simple as a banana and a glass of milk, or a handful of nuts. Stop whatever you are doing, though, to eat it slowly and savor it, even if you are at your desk.

Lunch should combine protein and bulk. A big salad with tuna and egg, home-made mayonnaise and home-made croutons, is a good example. Eat slowly. Chew well.

Mid afternoon snack could be sliced apple and cheese, or a small bunch of grapes, or add a few nuts. It is often a time when you start to flag, so a fructose boost from fruit works well.

Supper should ideally be early evening, or at *least* two hours before bedtime. Again, protein and not too heavy on the carbs—your digestion is on a 24-hour clock but don't overload it.

Late night snack is not essential, and if you don't feel remotely hungry, don't force yourself. However, if you are a bit of a night owl and it seems a long time since supper, a snack keeps your body nutritionally balanced while you are asking things of it. Cheese late at night can cause nightmares; generally avoid indigestible foods and try not to eat less than an hour before bedtime. It can be a treat, too. A strawberry smoothie with a teaspoon of honey? One or two squares of dark chocolate? Blueberries with Greek yogurt?

Chamomile tea will improve your sleep.

CHAPTER 5
Becoming more flexible through exercise

There are hundreds—*thousands*—of exercise books, videos, and routines. This chapter has a few tips, some general advice, and ten exercise suggestions.

When you're walking any kind of distance, bend your elbows and pump your arms for extra benefit.

Stretch before and after exercise.

Ten minutes of stretching every day, holding each position for ten seconds and not hurrying generally, will improve your flexibility one hundred-fold. Simple yoga stretches are the best for these.

While waiting for your bath to fill, swing your arms, do some knee-bends, twist your torso from side to side. Remember '*I must I must increase my bust, the more the better to fill my sweater*'? Very good for firming up the bust-line. Pull faces while you're doing your simple exercises. It isn't a workout as such, but it quickens your blood and feels surprisingly good.

Gardening is great but it is nearly impossible to set a regular regime of lifting, bending and stretching from one session to the next. It can't be your only exercise and anyway you'll enjoy it more, and manage more, if you are generally fit.

Doing more exercise does not automatically improve your health or slow down aging. In fact, it can have the opposite effect, putting unnecessary strain on your system. Work smarter, not harder.

Resistance training takes less time, and delivers better results. Water-based exercise, for one example, is *twice* as effective as the same movements on land.

Slow down your strength-training exercise moves, and hold for seconds longer, for maximum benefit.

Take a hot bath following a workout (or a strenuous gardening session) to improve circulation and ease off any residual soreness.

Social exercise will challenge you more than exercising alone, and is more fun. Walk with a friend, join an exercise group (yoga, Zumba, line-dancing), play tennis or lawn bowls.

Swedish massage, especially after exercise, is excellent for reducing inflammation, and muscle improvement.

Which exercise interests you?

1. Yoga isn't intensive, but it is very body-friendly. The stretches, smooth moves and unhurried action make it a stress-buster, along with improving muscle tone and flexibility.

2. Walking has the obvious advantage of ever-changing scenery. Borrow a dog, if you don't have your own, and roam. It is a great stress reliever into the bargain.

3. Power-walking (pumping your arms and speeding almost to jogging pace, but with one foot always on the ground, unlike running, where you leave the ground mid-stride) is considered by some to be more effective than either jogging or running for muscle tone. It is also lower impact, so there is less chance of injury or joint strain.

4. Swimming, if you have joint problems but want to build muscle tone, is excellent. Chances are the local pool will be advertising a water-based exercise class, too.

5. Zumba, line, swing, country, belly and ballroom dancing are all fun, sociable, and boost your enjoyment levels.

6. On the subject of dancing, teach yourself a stripper routine. There are YouTube tutorials, and you may find yourself laughing breathlessly more than dancing, but stripping routines (you can keep your clothes on!) are intricate and intensive, difficult to learn, and intriguing. Warm up well first.

7. Housework, or clearing the shed or garage, is a good time to put on dance music and dance while you work, adding an element of lightness to a chore.

8. Cycling can be the serious stuff in the full kit, or fitting a basket to the handlebars and cycling to the shops.

9. Martial arts – there are many types, and you can progress at your own pace, become ambitious or just enjoy the mental balance and physical confidence that comes with mastering even the basic moves.

10. An astonishing number of couples are finding that sex after menopause is in fact the best it has ever been. Something for younger readers to look forward to.

CHAPTER 6
Useful additives and herbal supplements

The healthiest dietary regime in the world would include everything you needed, but few of us can achieve that. There are so many herbal supplements and additives on offer that we would all rattle like pill-bottles if we took them all, not to mention having the most expensive pee in the world.

- Vitamin C is particularly good for older skin, and good for boosting the immune system.

- Cod's liver oil capsules keep joints supple and flexible.

- Echinacea throughout the winter will boost the immune system and help protect against colds and 'flu

For sleeping difficulties:

St John's Wort is good for depression-related mood and sleep disorders. The only disadvantage is that it must be taken over time for best results, as it has a cumulative effect. If you have chronic sleeplessness it is a real help, but if you have an occasional bad night it won't work as a one-step solution. (It also can't be taken if you are on the Pill, as they don't interact well.)

Bach remedies have the advantage of being easy to take, quick-acting, non-addictive and not too soporific. This makes them ideal if you realize at three in the morning that you aren't going to get back to sleep naturally. A few drops will relax you and soothe you back to sleep, unlike a sleeping pill, which will knock out most of the following day.

Also consider:

Some people swear by general-purpose multi-vitamins as an overall boost. Others insist Selenium is a must, as it is a potent antioxidant and repairs tissue damage. As long as you don't get yourself into that rattling-when-you-walk situation because you are taking so many extras, go with what works for you. However, keep it down; no more than five a day. A healthy diet covers nearly all the bases.

Although calcium is recommended as one gets older, it should always be taken in moderation, as it has side-effects including gas, constipation, confusion, kidney stones and muscle weakness. If you include enough dairy in your daily diet, you shouldn't need more than a tablet a week unless specifically advised by your doctor.

If you have a genetic history of kidney stones, a daily tablespoon of apple cider vinegar is a good idea. It is also effective if you have a tendency to those sudden agonizing leg cramps which seem to appear more often as we get older.

Don't forget to buy that eye-bath at the drugstore, and rinse your eyes regularly.

CONCLUSION
A sound mind in a healthy body

A healthy diet is a huge first step in maintaining mental acuity, exercise drives oxygen to the brain, and sufficient sleep adds quality to your waking hours.

Now that you are going to be looking good, eating well, and walking with a spring in your step, the last and most important step is to ensure you'll be enjoying the quality you have added to your life. Mental agility, good memory and general alertness are genetic gifts, but there are exercises even for the brain.

Avoid frustration and stress by avoiding contentious issues, especially if they don't directly concern you. Stop watching the world news if it frustrates or upsets you, just keep up with the headlines. However, read local magazines and newspapers and keep up with local issues.

If you use social media (Facebook, Twitter, etc.,) don't follow every link that presents itself. There is a growing belief that story-hopping is accelerating mental confusion and reducing our ability to concentrate. Ask yourself if you really want to know or are just mildly interested. Only follow the link if you really want to know. Reduce the time you spend on your social media to an hour at most.

Read for pleasure. There are millions of novels out there, join a book-club or re-read old favourites to get back into it if you no longer read much. Reading is relaxing, but also excellent for engaging concentration. Cozy whodunits are ideal light entertainment as they reward concentration if you can solve the mystery before the end.

Do crosswords, and mental agility tests like Sudoku. Play cards, even solitaire. Bridge players seem to keep mental acuity longer than anyone else. Board games like chess and draughts will stretch your brain. For that matter, any game that requires concentration and logic is good for you, and thanks to the internet you can pit yourself against players all over the world.

Learn a new language, or learn to play a musical instrument.

Watch intelligent quiz programs on television. Don't leave the television on in the background; only switch it on to watch a favourite show, as the constant background distraction does lead to mental confusion and the inability to concentrate.

Find old favourite songs on the internet, and enjoy the nostalgia. Songs (like smells) are powerful memory triggers and bring back happy times.

Smile.

Thank you again for downloading this book!

I hope this book was able to help you to live life to the fullest.

The next step is to get to work. And every day, in every way, get better and better.

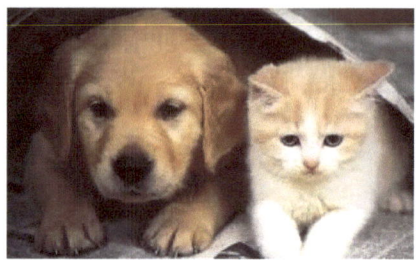

Finally, if you enjoyed this book, then I'd like to ask you for a favor, would you be kind enough to leave a review for this book on Amazon? It'd be greatly appreciated!

Thank you and good luck!

Preview Of My New Book

Crystals And Healing Stones: A Beginners Guide To Crystals Their Uses And Healing Power

For thousands of years, crystals have held a sacred and honored place among those who seek spiritual enlightenment, transformation, peace, and power. With this book, you're going to get a quick look at some of the more common crystals that you'll find at any local crystal shop and what they represent to those looking to do chakra work, meditation, or just carry them with them.

There are limitless possibilities when it comes to crystals and the power they provide. Let this book be the first step on an adventure of a lifetime as you experiment and study the unseen truths of the world. Watch your life transform through the power and energy of crystals and see what secrets you can unlock.

More Books by Michele Gilbert

Below you'll find some of my other books that are popular on Amazon and Kindle Simply click on the links below to check them out.

Stop Playing Mind Games: How To Free Yourself Of Controlling And Manipulating Relationships

Instant Charisma: A Quick And Easy Guide To Talk, Impress, And Make Anyone Like You

Chakras: Understanding The 7 Main Chakras For Beginners: The Ultimate Guide To Chakra Mindfulness, Balance and Healing

Practicing Mindfulness: Living in the moment through Meditation: Everyday Habits and Rituals to help you achieve inner peace

Sleep Tight: Overcome Insomnia and Sleep Disorders for a better more restful sleep!

Stop Back Pain Now!: Back Pain Remedies and Treatments so you can live a pain free life!

The Arthritis Pain Cure: How to find Arthritis Pain Relief and live a happy pain free life!

The Headache Pain Cure: How to find Headache Pain Relief and live a happy Pain Free Life!

Stop Panic Attacks and Anxiety Disorders without Drugs Now!: Overcome Panic, Stress and Anxiety and live a happy pain free life!

The Breakup Recovery Guide: Advice for Surviving Heartbreak, Letting Go and Thriving in an exciting new life!

The Friendship Guide to Finding Friends Forever: How to Find, Make and Keep Quality Friendships After your Breakup

The Credit Fix: Leave behind credit card debt and poor credit scores and get your life back!

How To Stop Being Jealous And Insecure: Overcome Insecurity And Relationship Jealousy

www.ingramcontent.com/pod-product-compliance
Lightning Source LLC
Chambersburg PA
CBHW050928290526
45792CB00002B/932